MY LOVELY DENTIST MANDALA COLORING BOOK

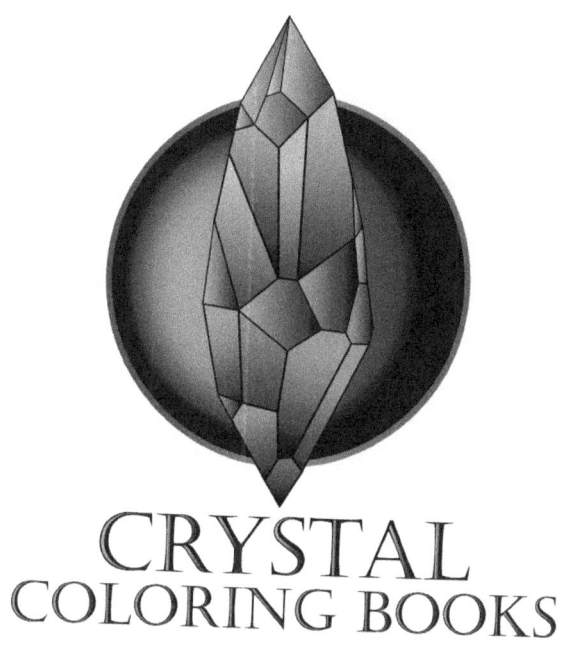

CRYSTAL COLORING BOOKS

Copyright © 2018 Crystal Coloring Books
All rights reserved.

ISBN-13: 978-1719481861
ISBN-10: 1719481865

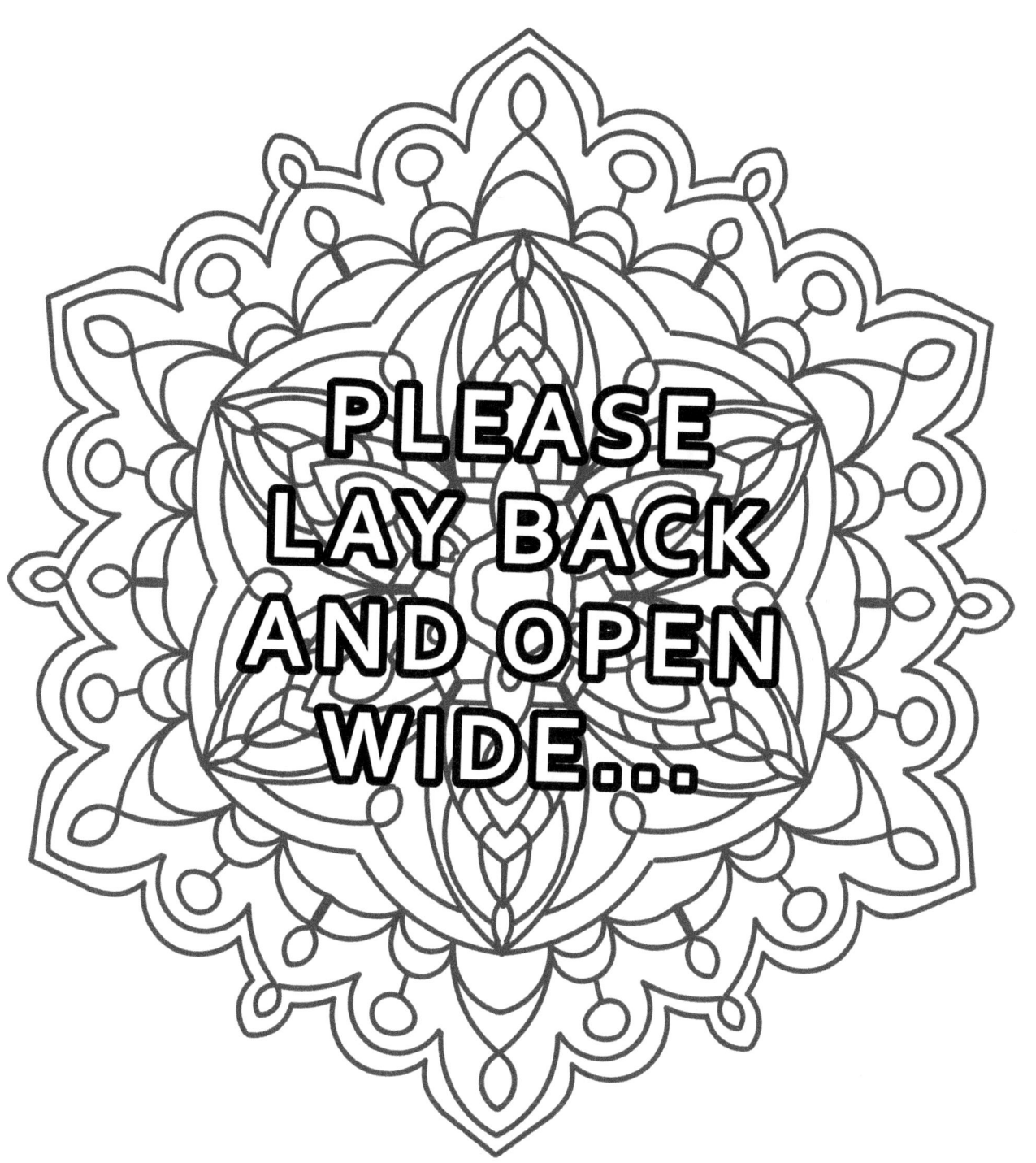

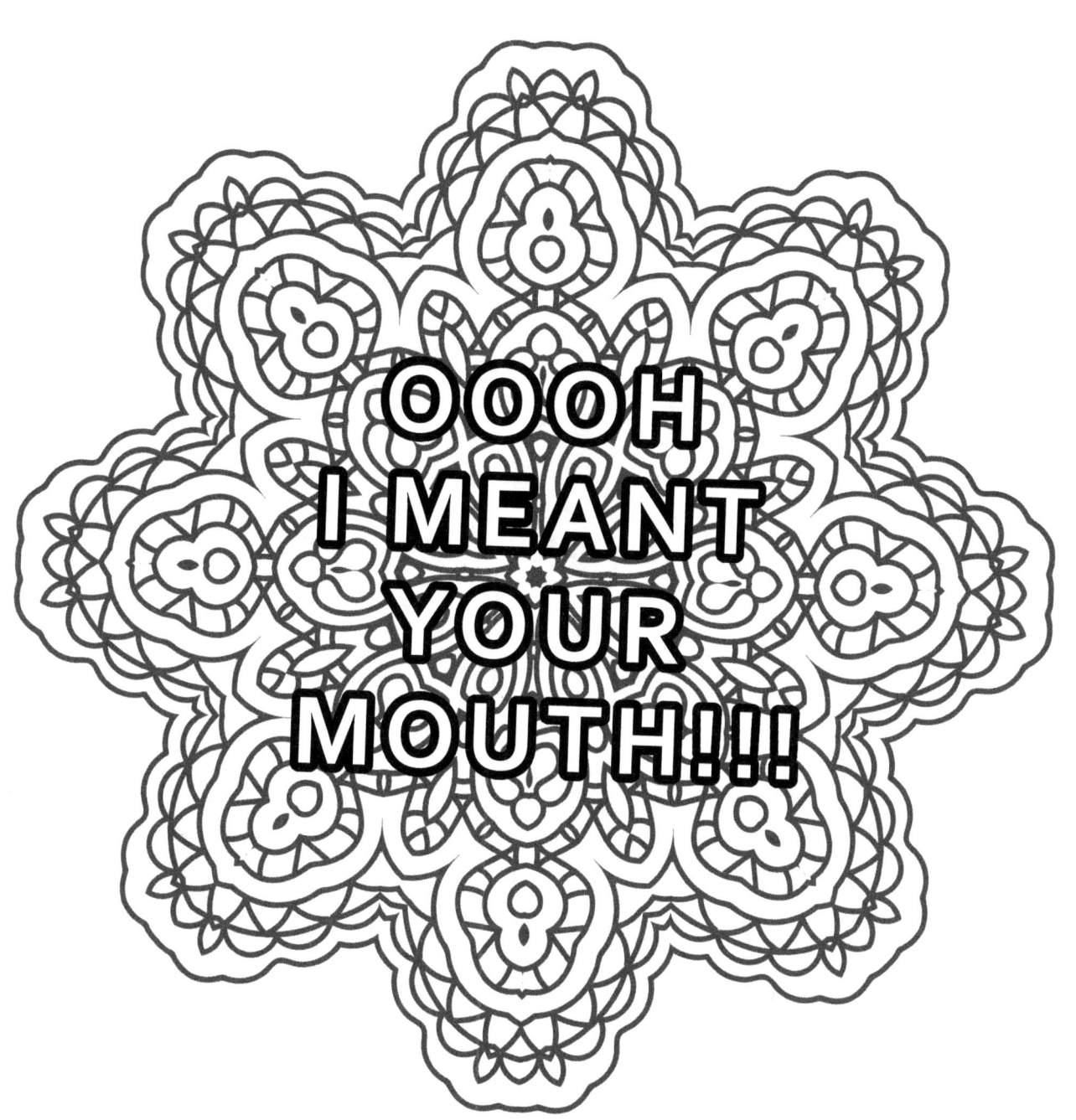

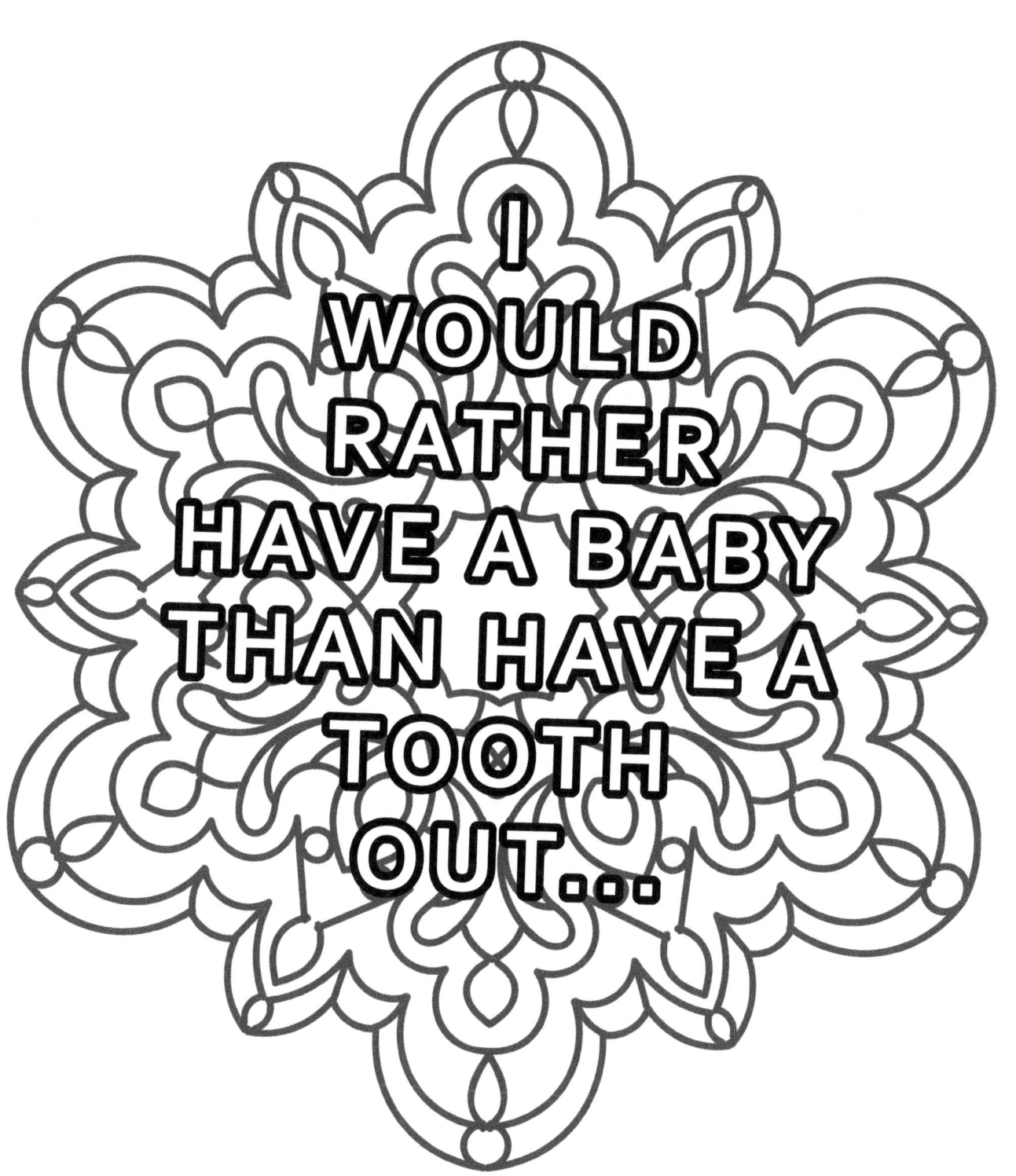

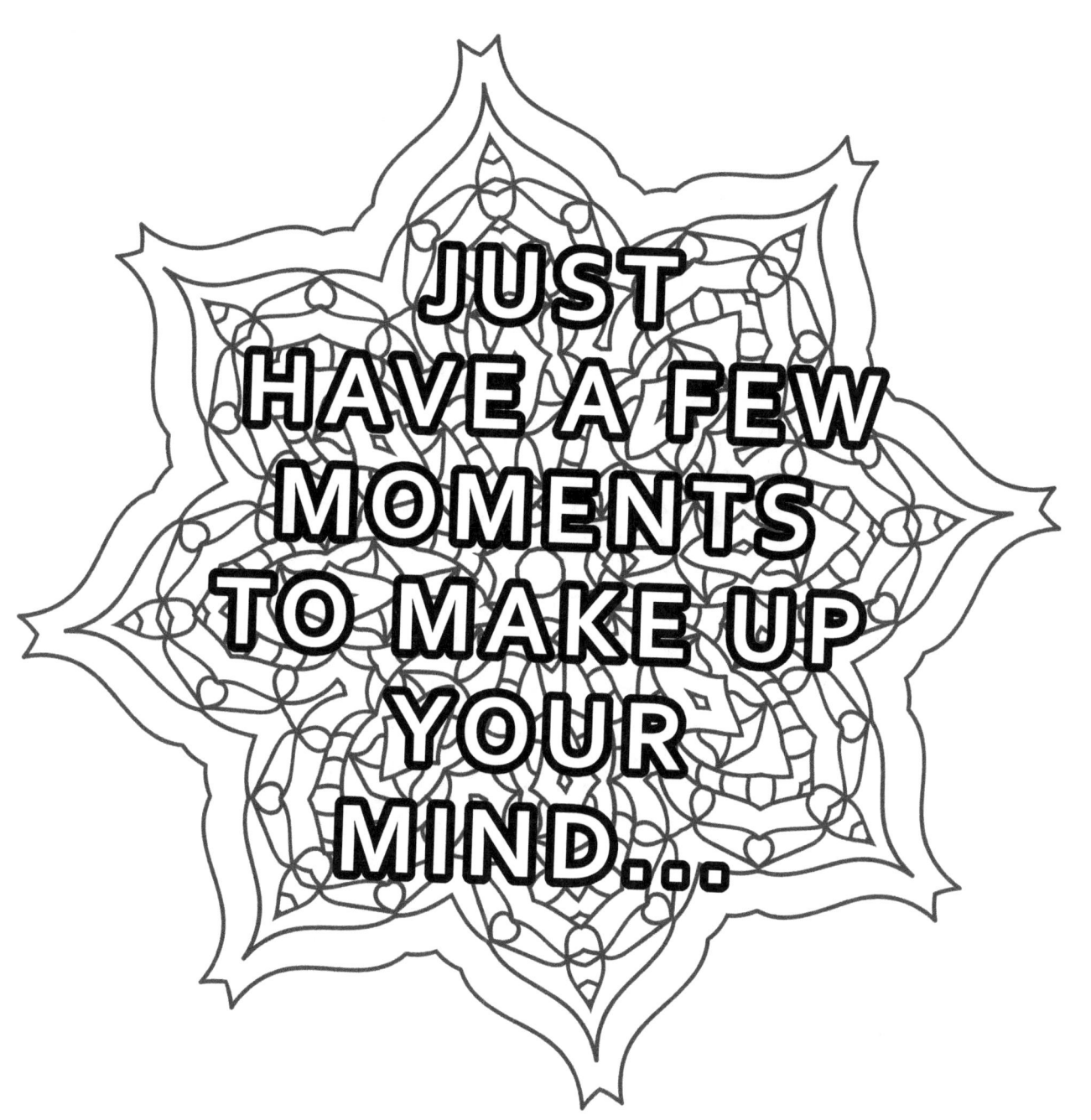

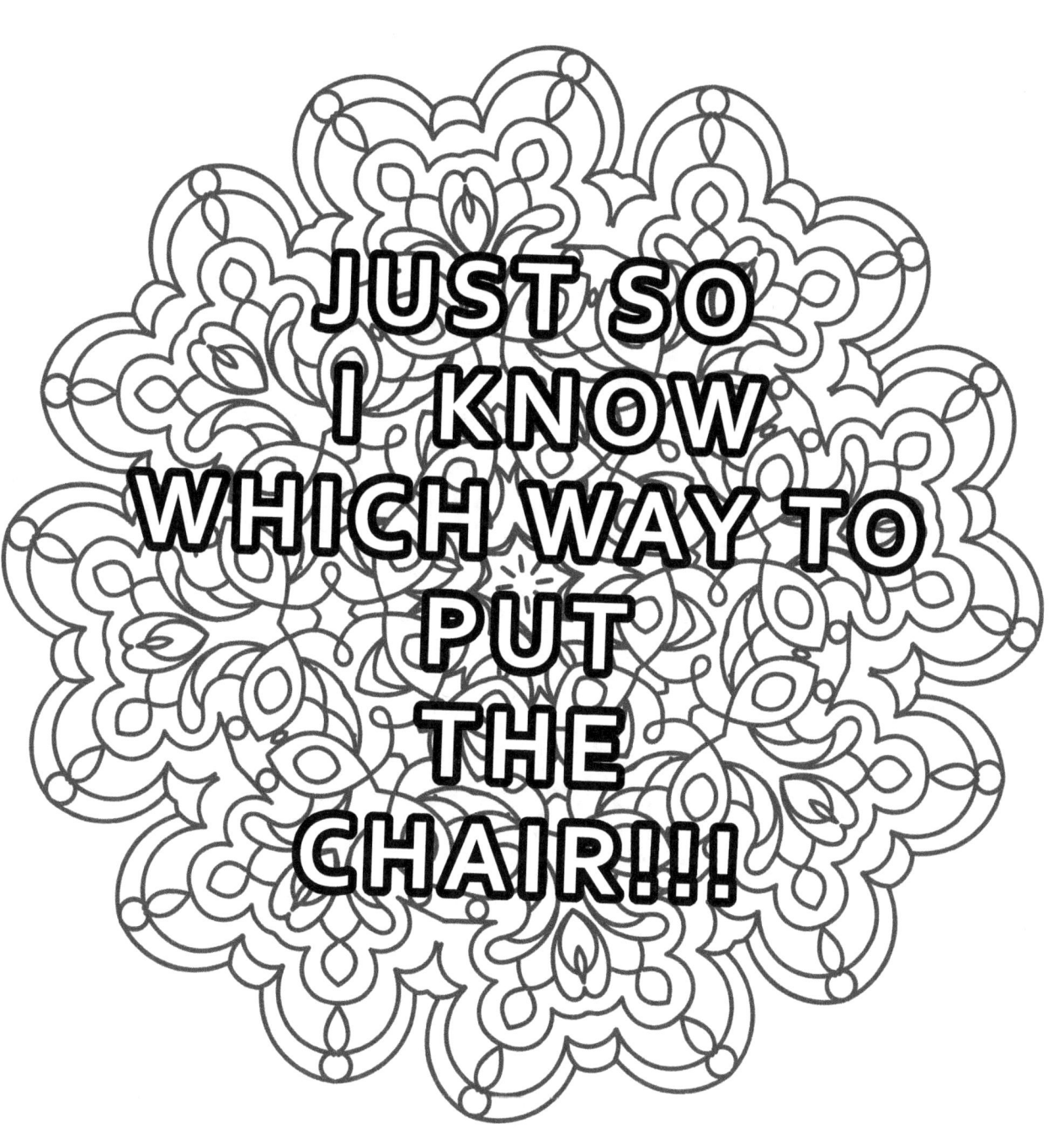

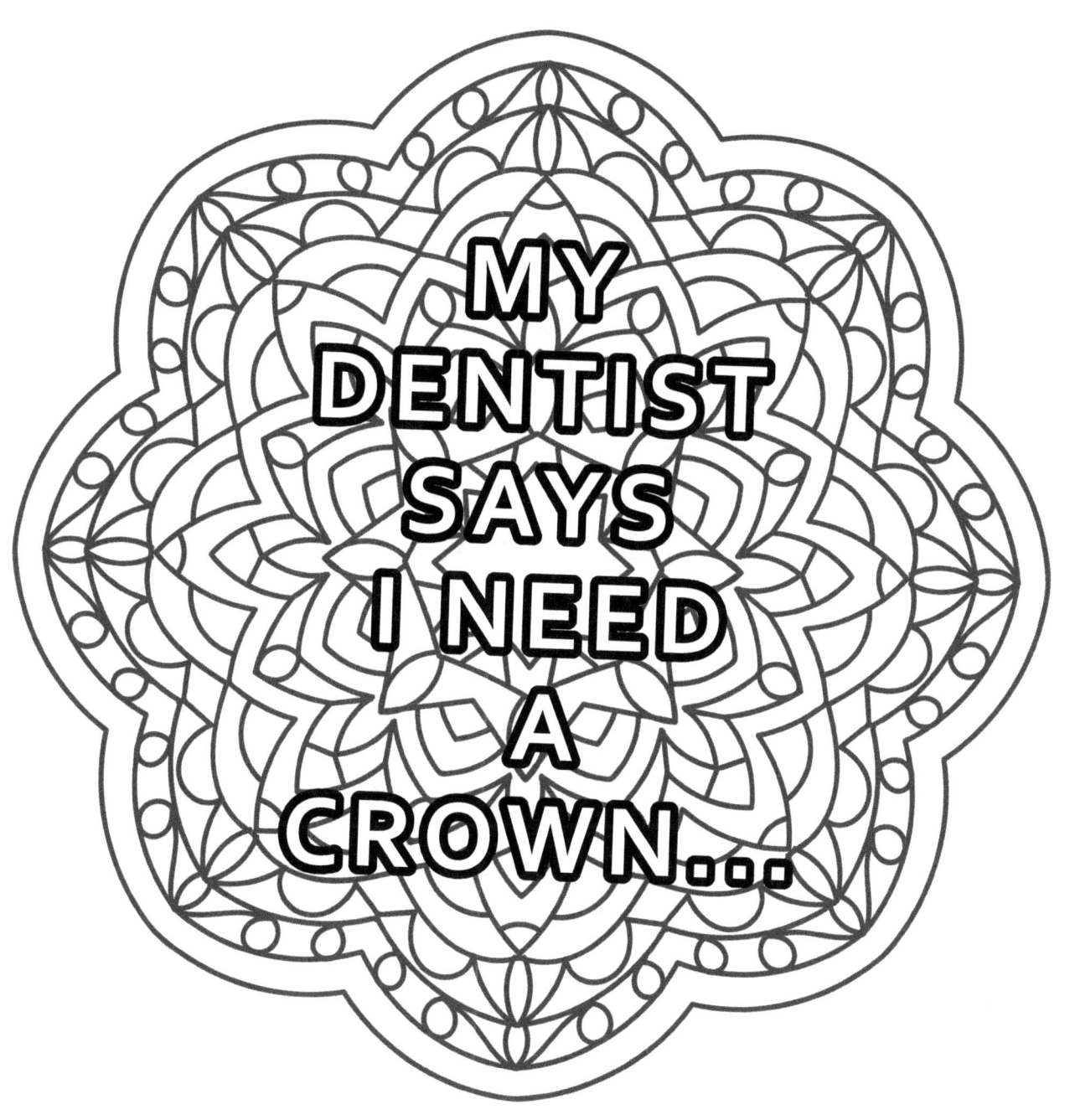

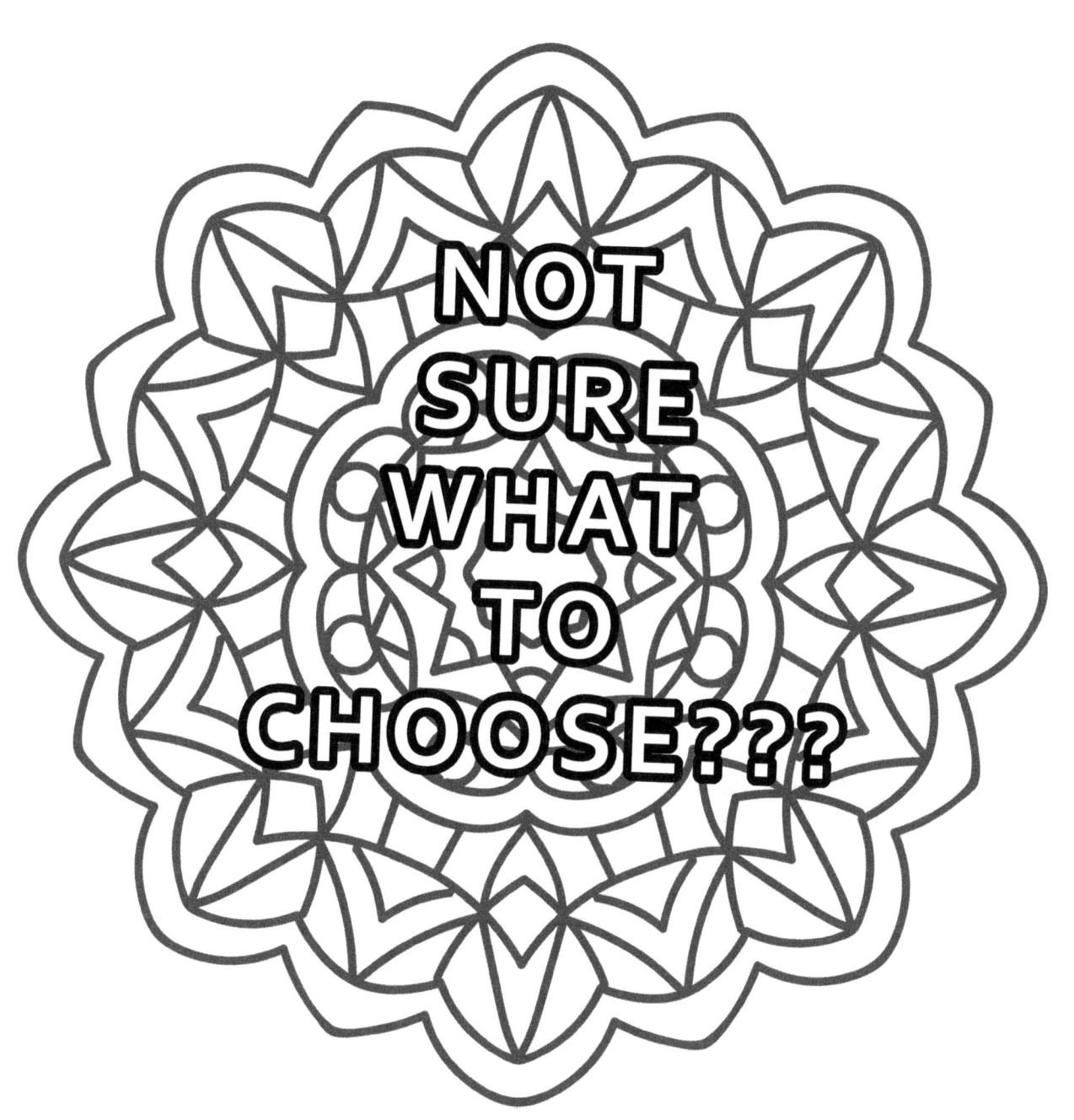

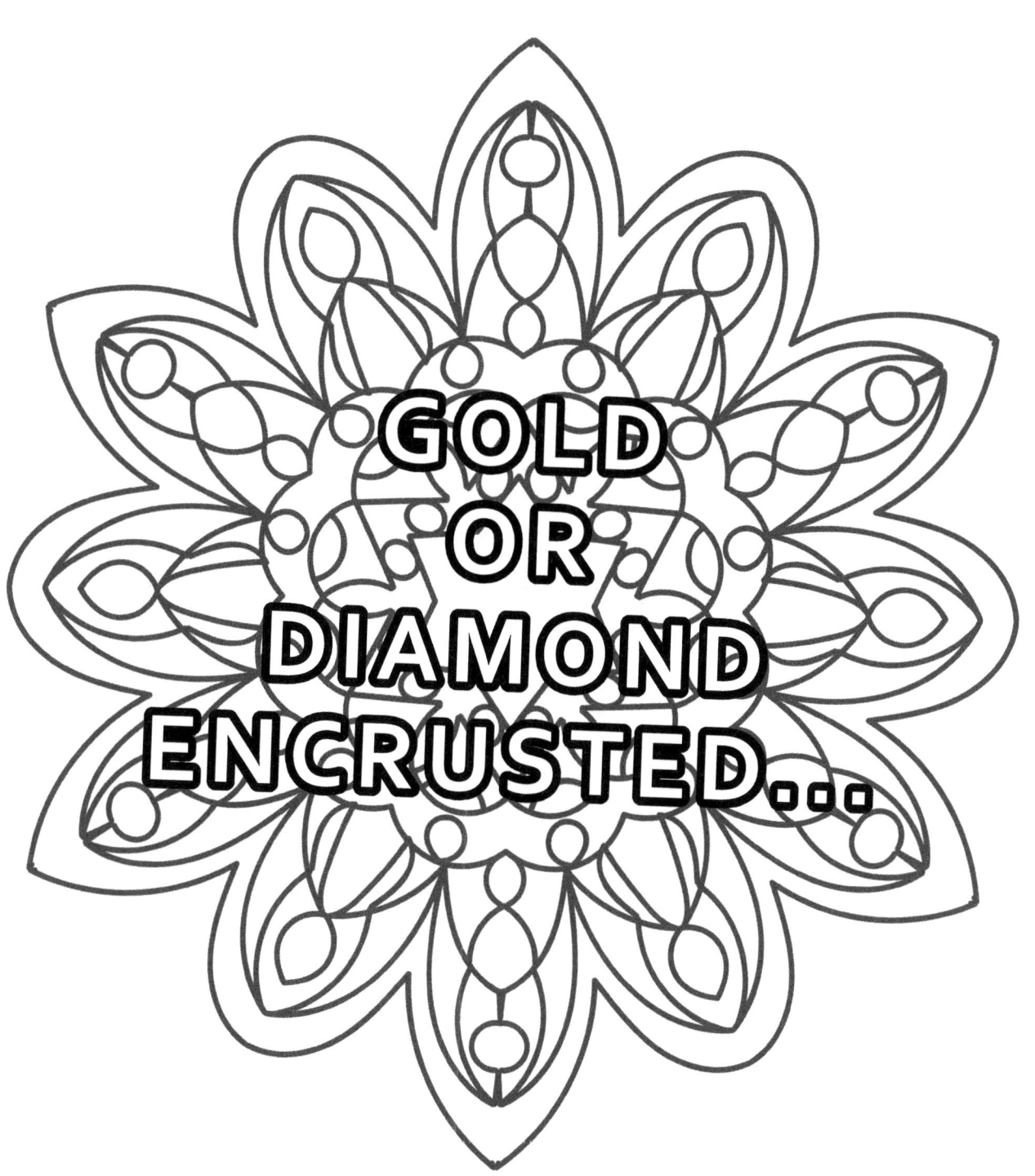

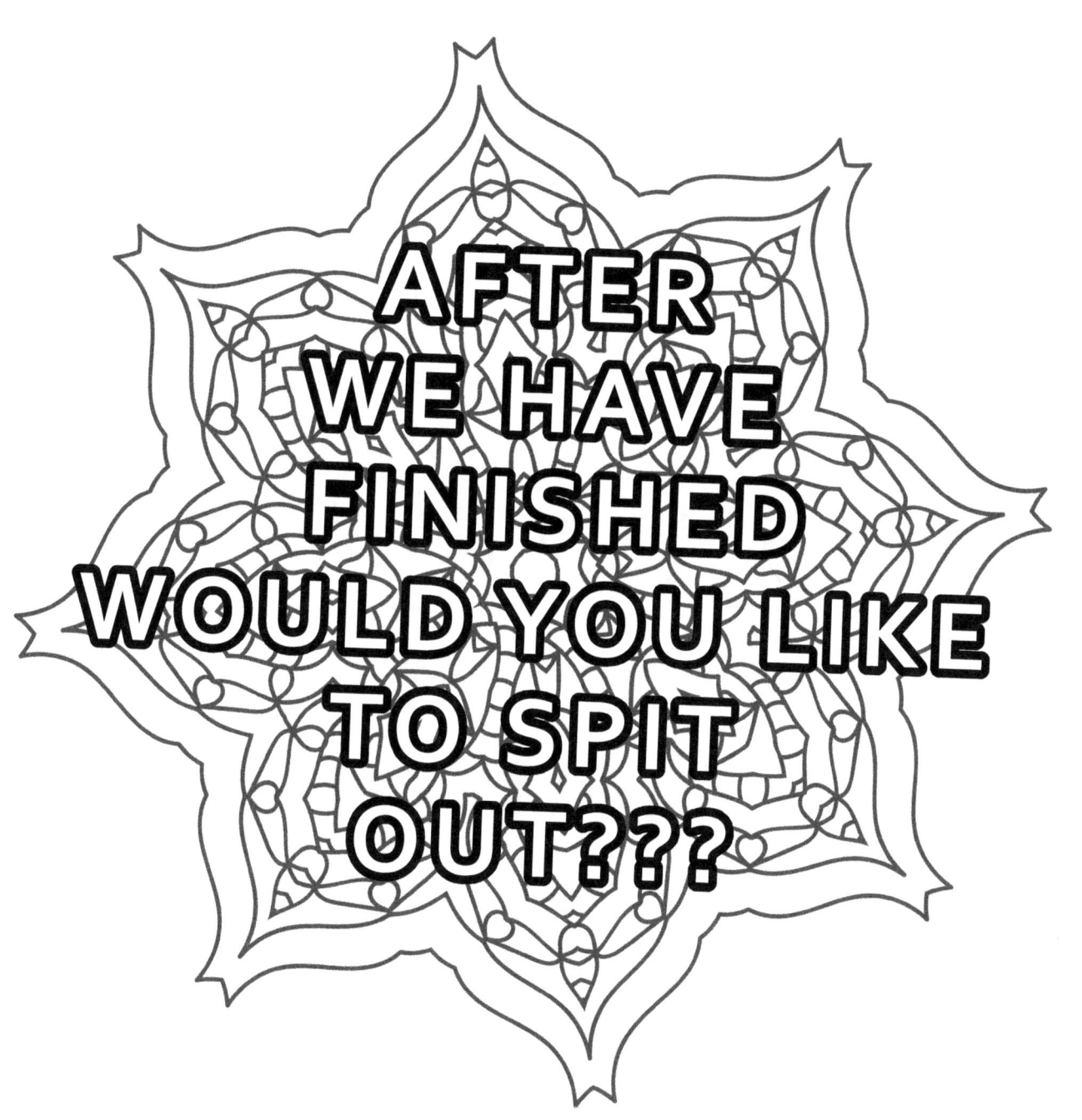

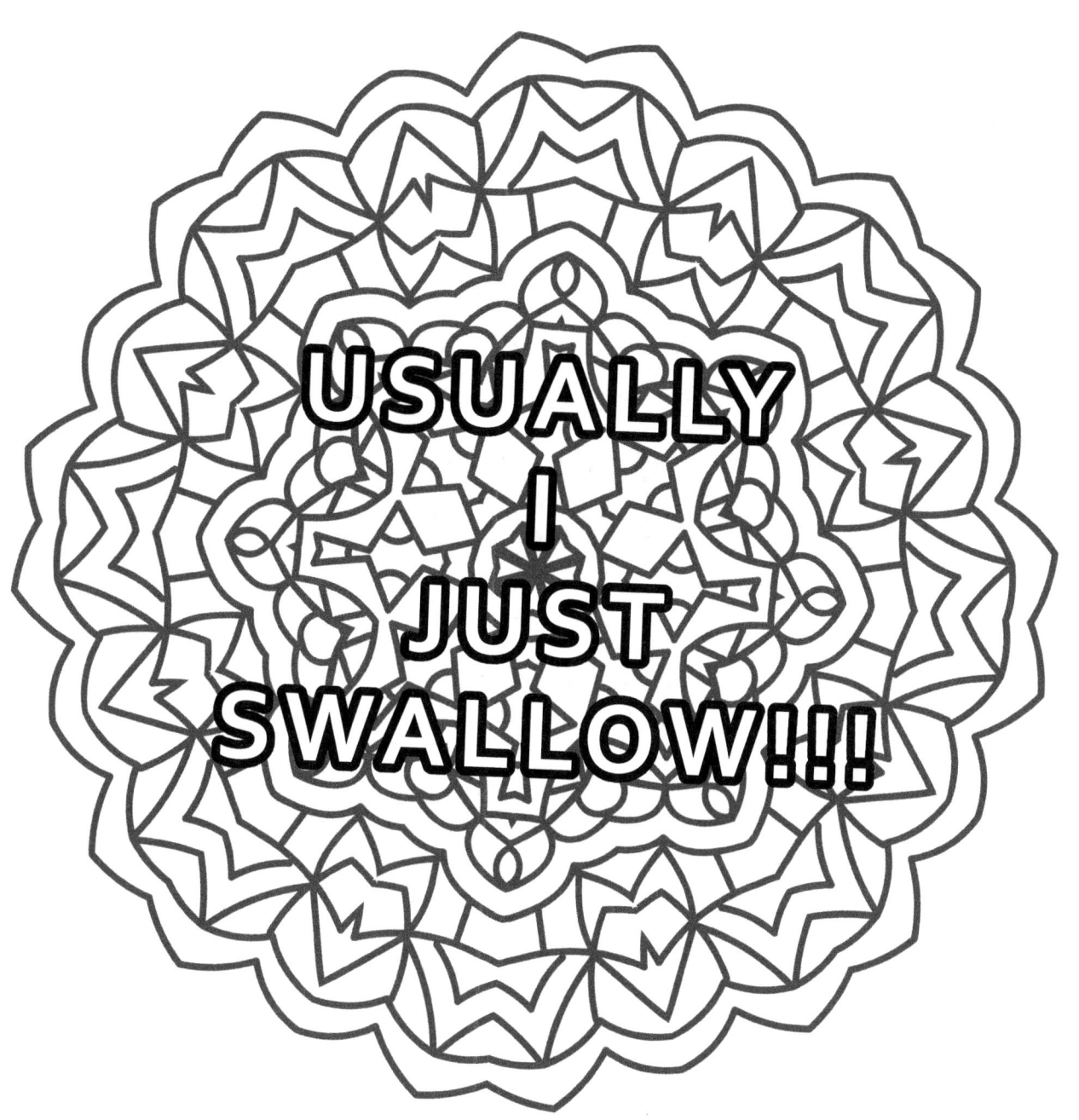

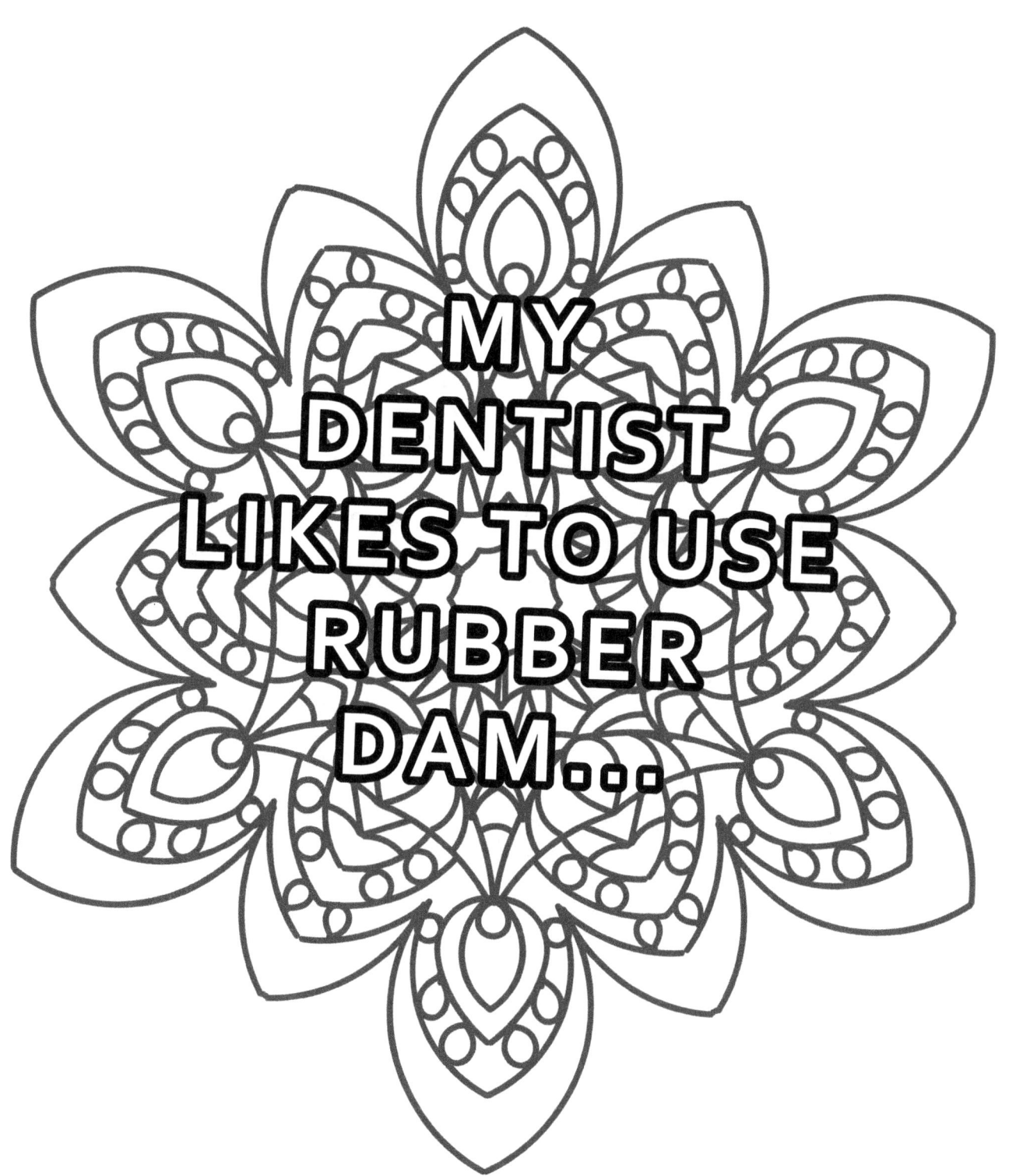

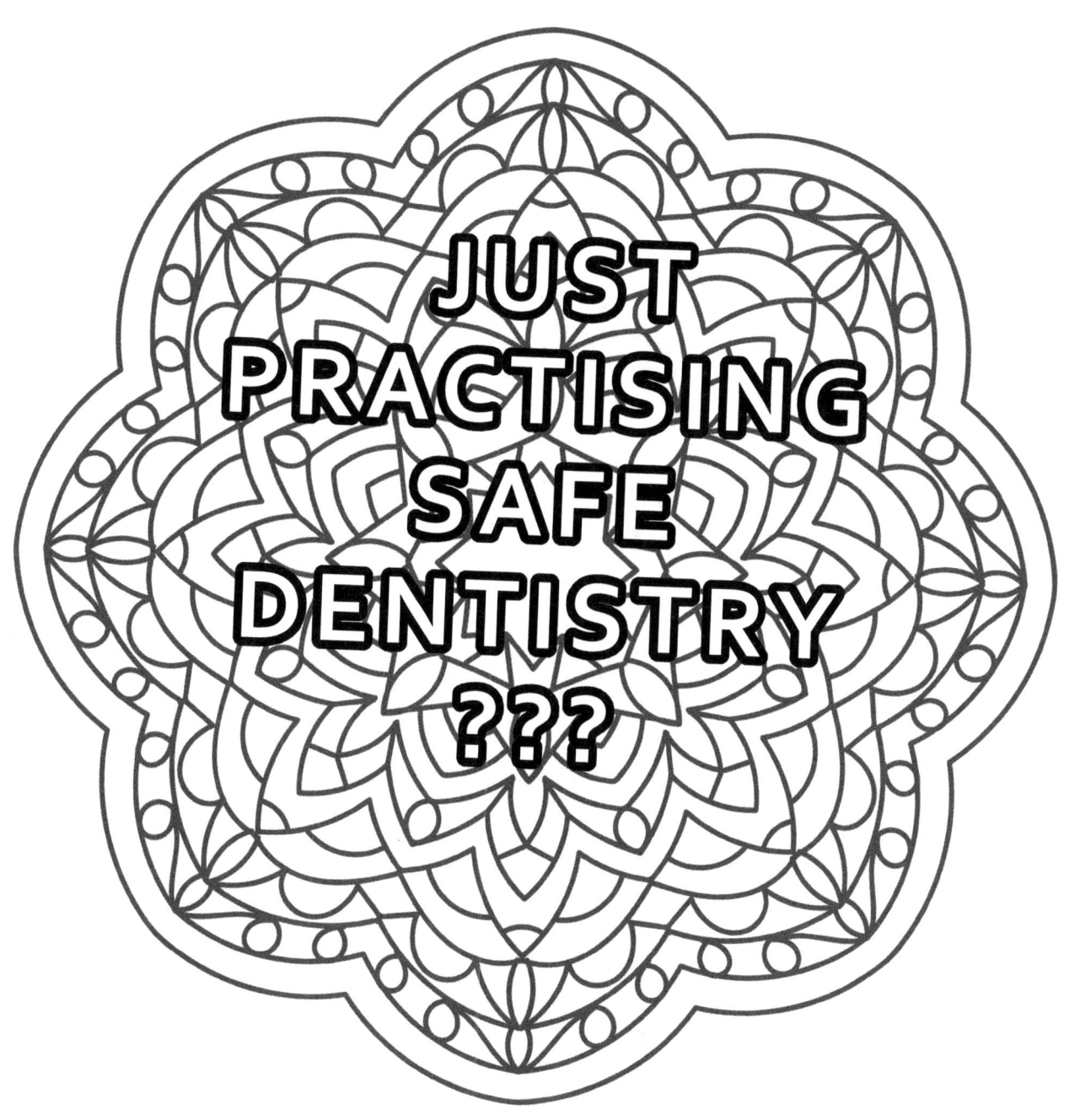

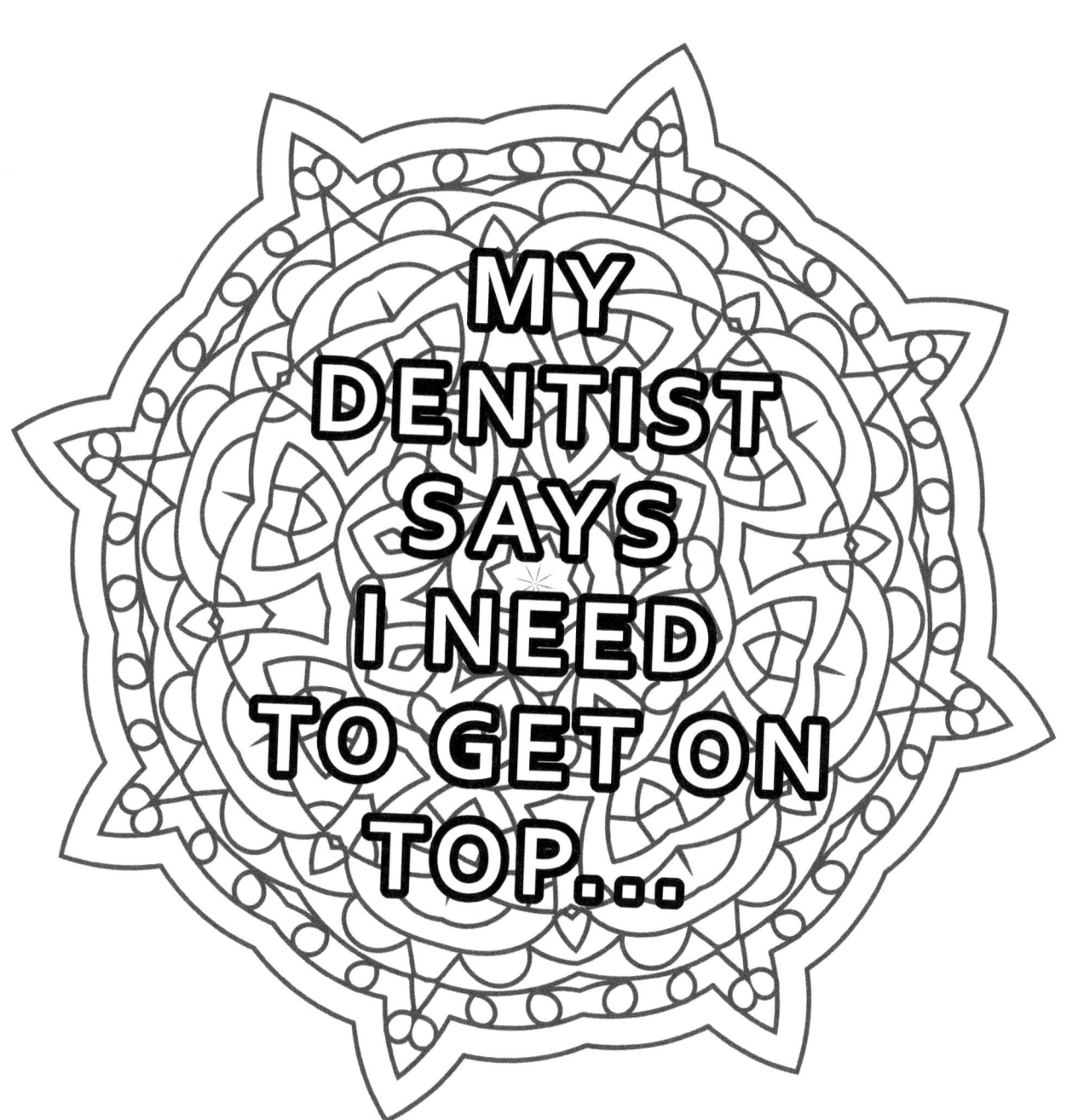

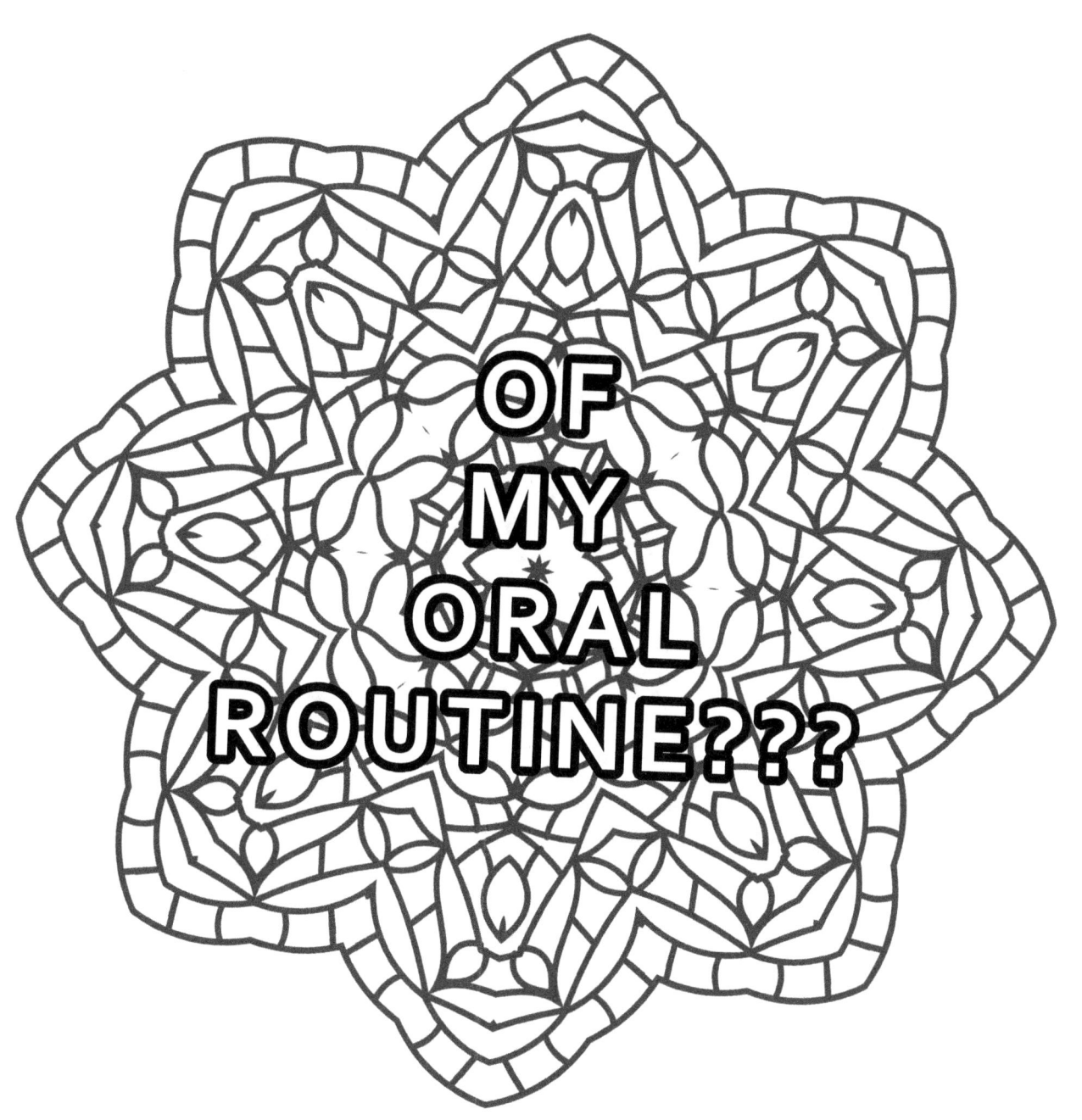

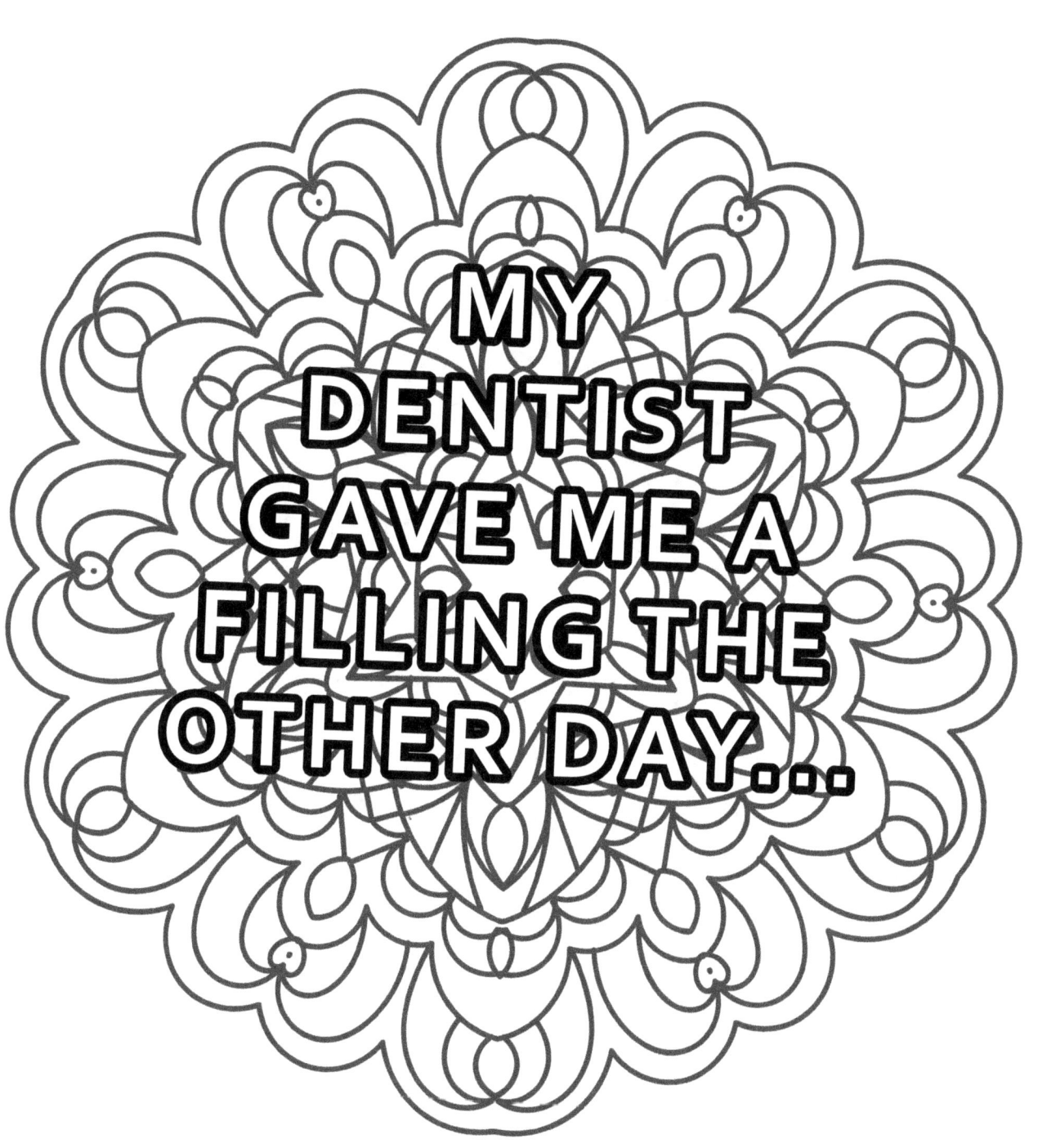

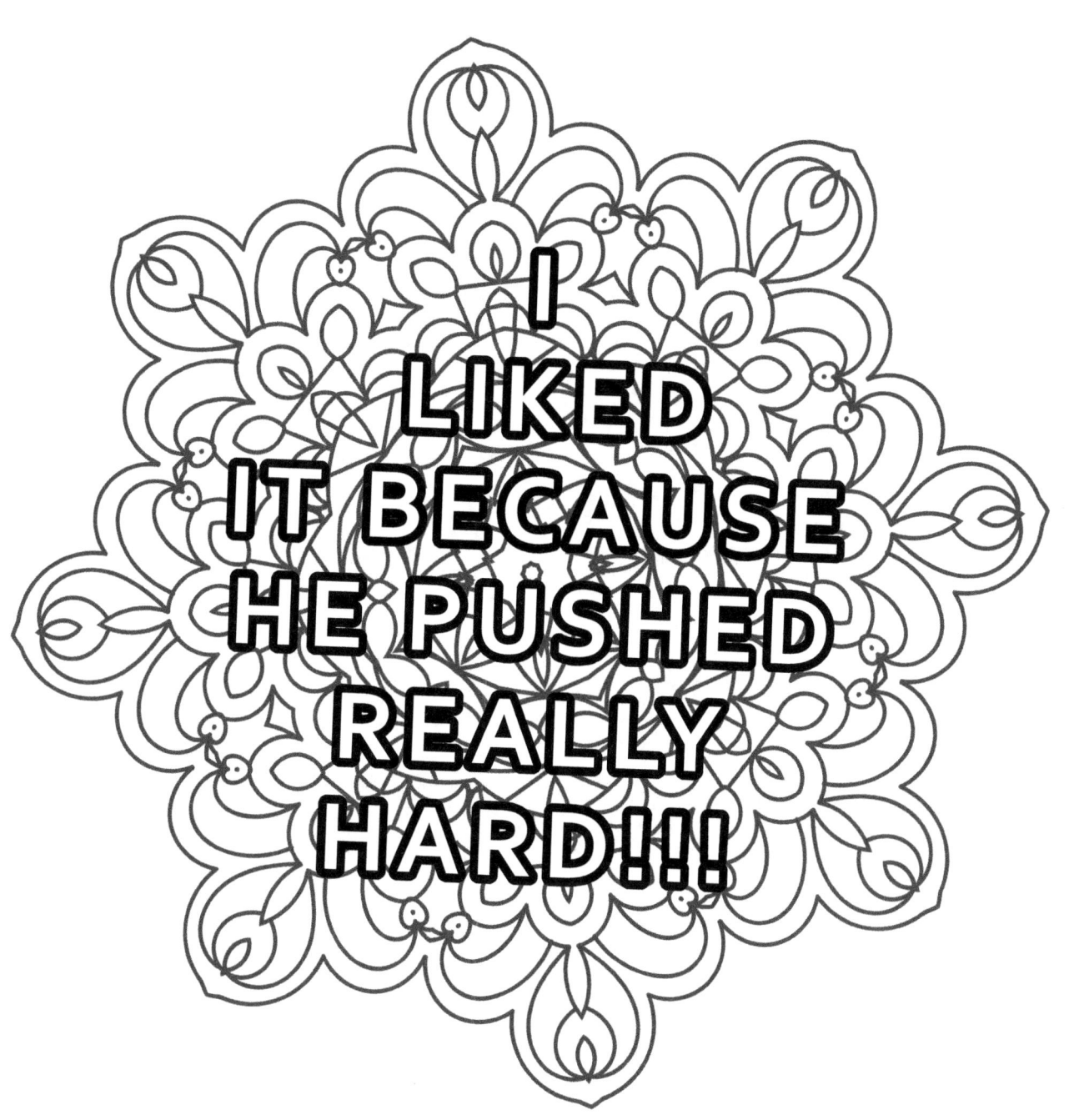

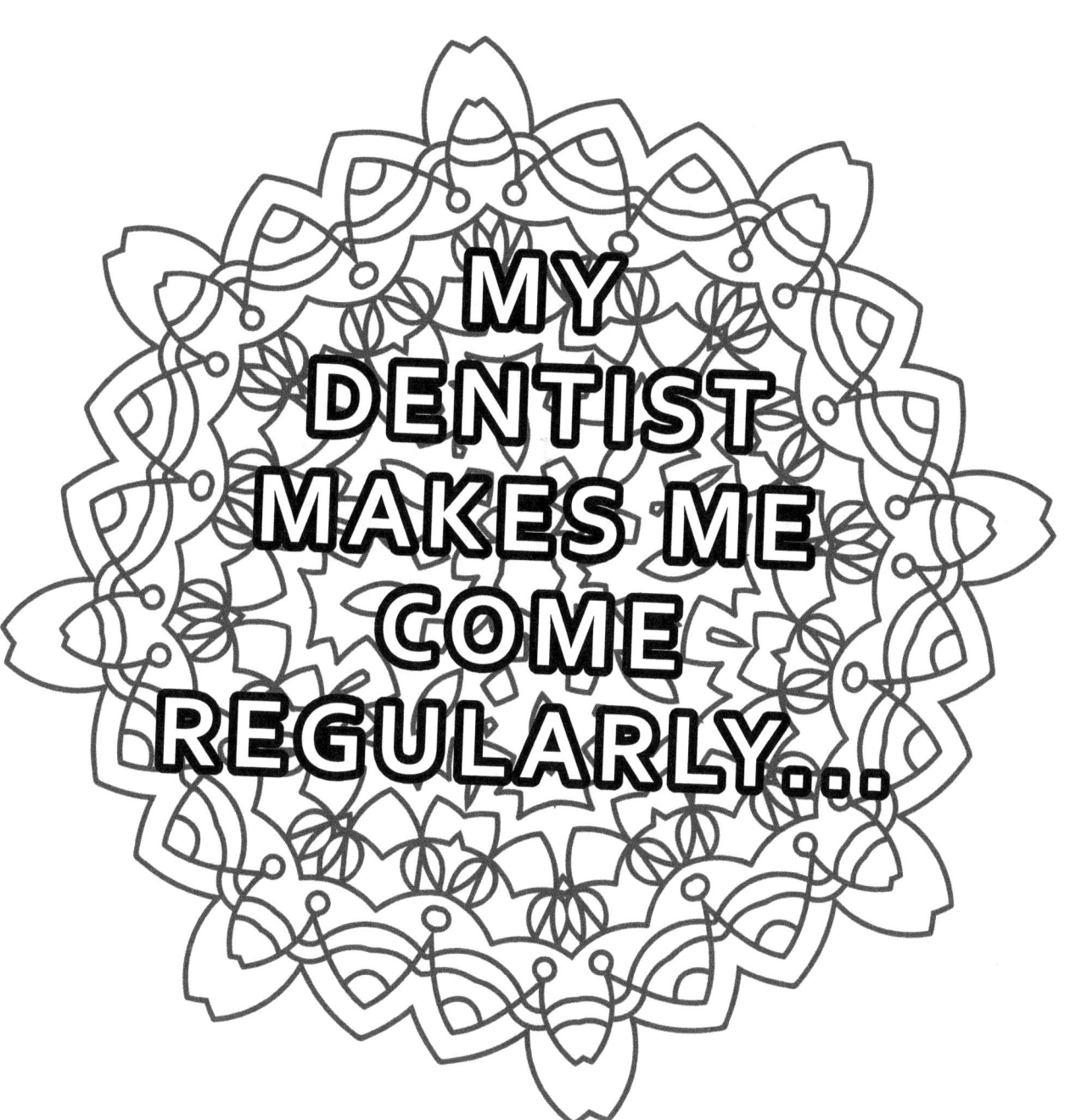

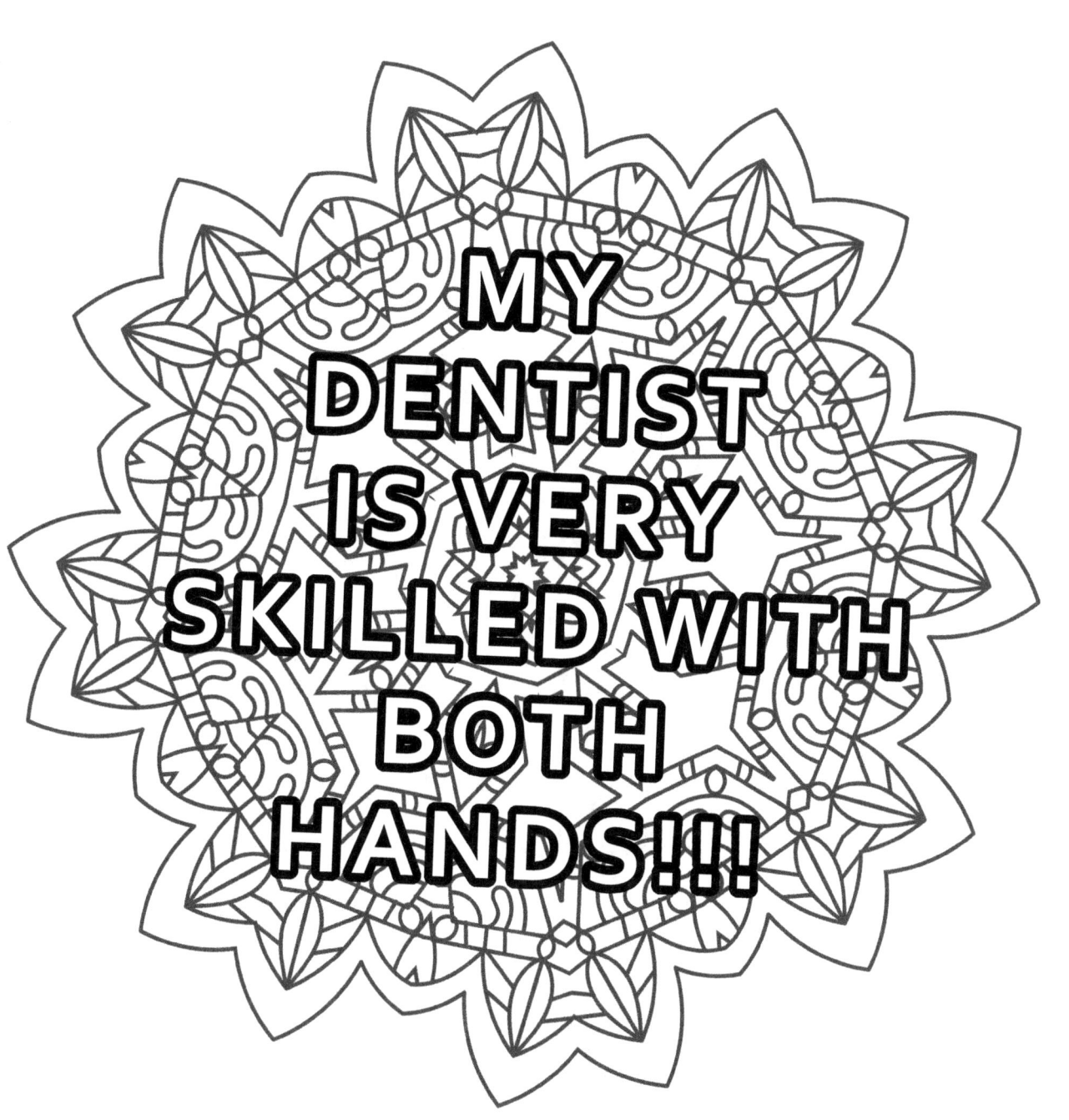

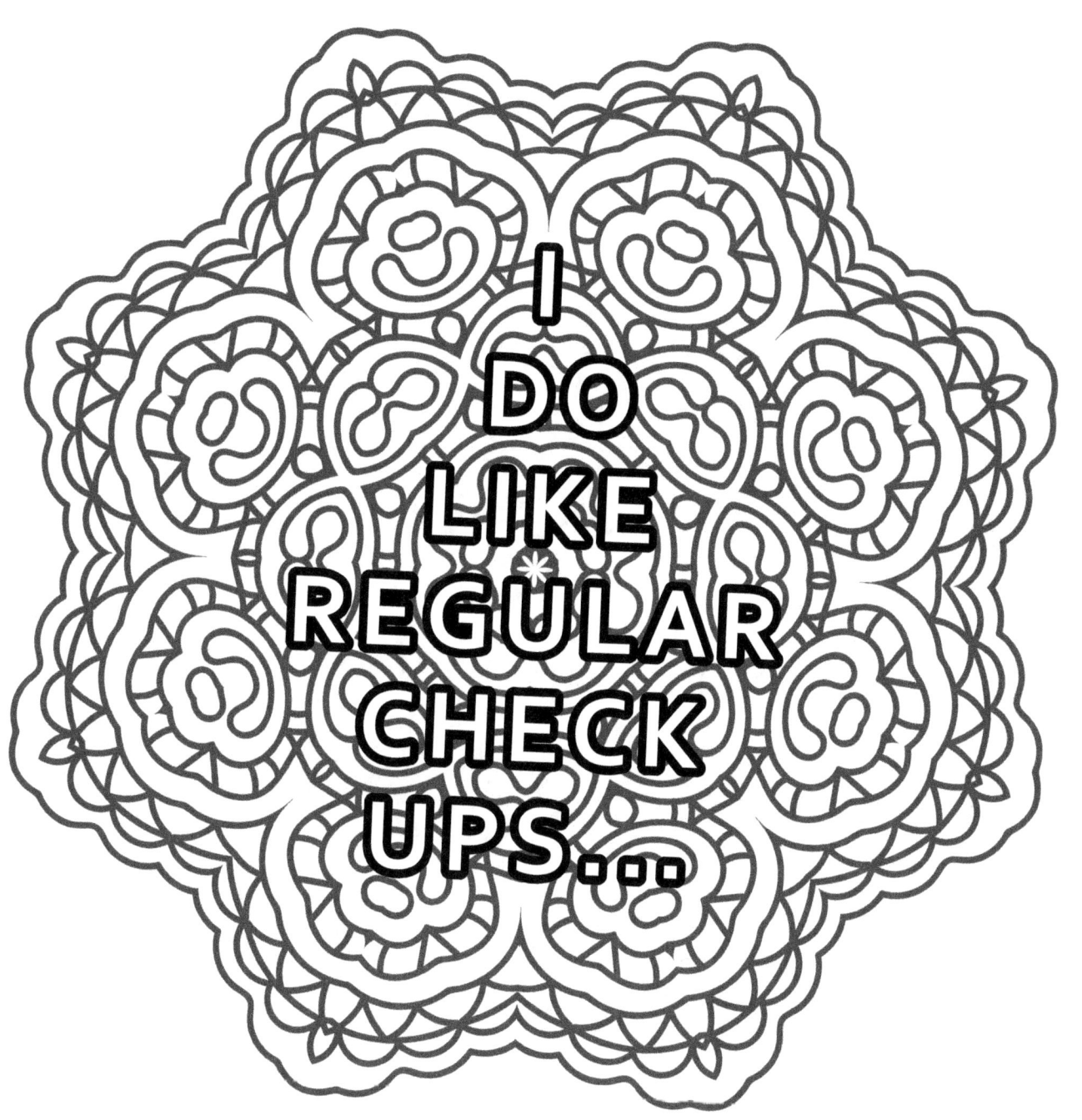

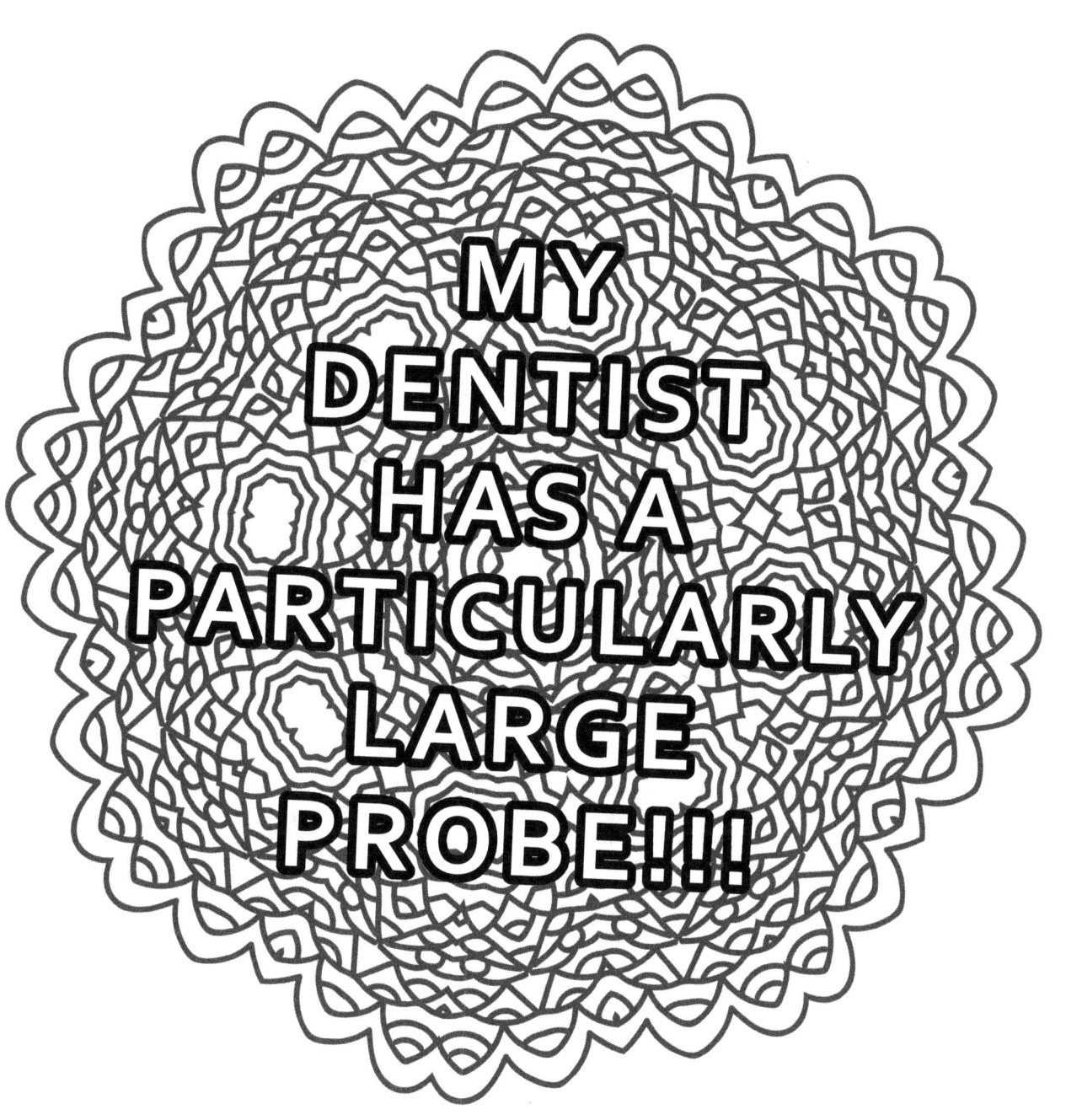

COLOR TEST PAGE

www.ingramcontent.com/pod-product-compliance
Lightning Source LLC
Chambersburg PA
CBHW082123220526
45472CB00009B/2282